I HAVE A FRIEND
WHO IS DEAF

HANNAH CARLSON, M. ED., CRC
DALE CARLSON

illustrated by
HOPE M. DOUGLAS, M.A.

CHANEY SHANNON PRESS
BICK PUBLISHING HOUSE
MADISON, CT

Text © copyright 1995 by Hannah Carlson, M. Ed., CRC
and Dale Carlson
© illustrations 1995 by Hope M. Douglas, M.A.
© cover and book design 1995 by Jane Miller Productions

Edited by Ann Maurer

With thanks to The Kennedy Center and
The National Theatre of the Deaf

CHANEY SHANNON PRESS is a trademark of
BICK PUBLISHING HOUSE

Library of Congress Catalog Card Number: 95-79844

ISBN: 1-884158-08-0--Volume 3
ISBN: 1-884158-11-0 --4-Volume Set

Printed by Royal Printing, Guilford, CT, USA

Special needs/disabilities

"These books are an important service. They are informed, practical guides to feelings, behavior patterns, medical facts, technology, and resources for people who care about people with disabilities."
>   –Richard Fucci, former president of the National Spinal Cord Injury Association

"Excellent, very informative."
>   –Alan R. Ecker, M.D., Assistant Clinical Professor of Opthalmology, Yale University

"An invaluable source of help and comfort for friends and caregivers of people who have disabilities or special needs."
>   –Mary Jon Edwards, Nationally Certified Therapeutic Horseback Riding Instructor, Special Olympics

"Excellent introductory handbooks about disabilities and special needs. They discuss medical conditions and rehabilitation, feelings and adaptive technology, and responsible attitudes both on the part of people with disabilities and people temporarily without them. The emphasis is on our common humanity, not our differences."
>   –Lynn McCrystal, M.ED.,vice-president, The Kennedy Center

"The books offer professional information in an easy-to-use, uncomplicated style."
>   –Renee Abbott, Group Home Director, S.A.R.A.H., Shoreline Association for the Retarded and Handicapped

"Precise information, good reading for the layperson."
>   –Jane Chamberlin, parent and employment supervisor, West Haven Community House

"Thank you for the opportunity to be a part of this work."
>   –Christine M. Gaglio, employment specialist for the deaf, The Kennedy Center

CONTENTS

NOTE

Disabilities are not necessarily the loss of the senses. It is more often society that disables, with its misinformation, prejudices, lack of understanding. What people call disabilities are invariably inconveniences, but rarely are people who have disabilities any more sick than anyone else. Yet too often a social death precedes a physical death in a world that regards a physical limitation as a failure and entertains a primitive fear that it is somehow catching.

The biggest problem people with deafness or hearing loss encounter is that of living in a world of sound, that insists on auditory cues, that treats those without hearing as if they were without sense.

If you are family or caregiver, old friend or new friend, learn that there are resources for information, help, and reassurance, and in a world that tends to avoid or misunderstand, an offer of help and knowledge of what is available can be an end to the despair of isolation.

ACKNOWLEDGMENTS

Our gratitude to Theodore Harold Bromm and Renee Abbott, Group Home Director, both of S.A.R.A.H., the Shoreline Association of the Retarded and Handicapped; to Richard Fucci, former president of the National Spinal Cord Injury Association; to Alan Ecker, M.D., Assistant Clinical Professor of Opthalmolgy at Yale University; to Jane Chamberlin, parent and employment supervisor, West Haven Community House; and to Lynn McCrystal, M.Ed., vice-president, The Kennedy Center, for their counsel and editorial advice.

Our gratitude to Louis and Susan Weady, not only for Royal Printing, but for their guidance and patience with new editions, purchase orders, and shipping.

Our special thanks to Herb Swartz for his kindness and the use of his computers.

Our further special thanks to Danny Carlson for teaching us how to use computer capabilities for publishing.

And our thanks to Terrence Finnegan for providing Bick Publishing House with its own computer system.

1

HAVING A HEARING LOSS: CONDITIONS

Some people are born with little or no ability to hear. Others develop hearing impairments during the course of their lives due to disease or injury. However the hearing loss occured, not being able to hear meaningful or even critical sounds can be isolating and sometimes frightening.

There are approximately 16 million Americans who have significant difficulty hearing. Two million of those people have been diagnosed as being deaf. Hearing loss varies from mild to profound.

Being deaf or hard of hearing is a very isolating experience. Because of their need to communicate with others, the hearing impaired have built up a complex and tightly-knit deaf culture that has evolved over centuries. This culture is taught and shared in special schools for the deaf, from primary and secondary schools to those that specialize in the arts or in business, and much else. The schools are conducted mostly through sign language. The deaf culture provides friendship, support, a sense of connectedness and identification with others in the community. They nurture and help others, and are themselves nurtured and helped to develop their own capacities.

Some people who are deaf or hard of hearing also have speech difficulties. This is particularly true of severe hearing losses that occur at birth where the child does not have the opportunity to hear proper speech production or articulation. Malformations at birth in the muscles or structure of the face can also interfere with a person's ability to speak.

It is important to remember that deafness is a separate problem. Most of the time it is an invisible problem. But there are some additional medical disorders that can accompany deafness or hearing loss. These include cerebral palsy, mental retardation, or attention deficit disorder.

CAUSES OF HEARING LOSS

Here is a partial list of conditions associated with hearing loss and deafness.

Prenatal – during pregnancy

1. inherited hearing loss or deafness through a parent's genes (deaf parents are more likely to have deaf children)

2. malformed ear canals, eardrums, or small bones in the middle ear (incus, stapes, malleus)

3. deformities in the sensory receptors of the inner ear(cochlea), auditory tract, or auditory centers of the brain

4. cranio-facial malformations involving the skull, face, nose, ears, or lips such as a cleft palate

5. environmental influences (malnutrition, poisons, drugs, maternal diseases such as Rubella, toxoplasmosis, herpes infections during pregnancy)

Perinatal – in and around labor and delivery

1. intrauterine disorders (abnormal labor and delivery, significant oxygen deprivation, respiratory difficulties just after birth)

2. neonatal disorders (intracranial hemorrhage, infections such as meningitis, head trauma at birth, jaundice at birth)

3. low birth weight (less than approximately three pounds)

Postnatal – after delivery
1. diseases that affect the auditory nerve or auditory centers of the brain (measles, mumps, chicken pox) repeated ear infections, or infections with a high fever

2. head injuries (accidents, abuse)

3. environmental influences (toxic effect of certain medications on the auditory cranial nerve)

4. excessive ear wax blocking the ear canal

5. repeated exposure to loud noises (rock concerts), close range

exposure to exploding sounds (bombs, explosives, gunfire).

Loud noise means:

a. having to raise your voice to be heard

b. not being able to hear someone less than two feet away talking

Signs your hearing may have been affected include:

a. speech sounding muffled or dull after the noise has ended

b. ringing or pain in ears after hearing the noise

6. progressive deterioration of hearing due to the natural aging process (called Presbycusis)

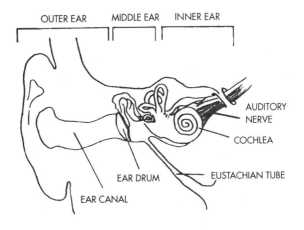

HEARING LOSS DEFINED

There are four types of hearing loss based on the nature and location of the injury.

Conductive

Diseases or obstructions to the outer or middle ear such as excessive ear wax or ear infections that produce fluid or swelling, and block sound to the inner ear, can cause hearing loss. Obstructions caused by malformed ear canals, eardrums, or small bones in the middle ear can result in permanent loss. Sounds are muffled, but not distorted. Usually, it does not result in a severe loss. People with this type of hearing loss benefit from hearing aids.

Sensorineural

Damage to the sensory hair cells of the inner ear cause hearing loss. Damage can come from childhood diseases, malformations in the inner ear, some medications, traumatic brain injury, or repeated trauma such as hearing loud noises for long periods of time. Sounds are distorted so that increasing the volume will not improve the quality. Hearing losses usually vary from mild to profound. Deafness can result from damage in this area.

Mixed

When both conductive and sensorineural impairments are present, that is, in the middle and outer ear, the hearing loss is called "mixed."

Central

Defects or damage to the auditory tracts of the central nervous system such as the auditory nerve (eighth cranial nerve, Vestibulocochlear) cause hearing loss. Damage can occur in the pathways leading to the brain or within the brain. Hearing loss can result from brain dysfunction present at birth, tumors, lesions (scars) of the central nervous system, strokes, or certain medications.

HEARING LOSS CLASSIFICATIONS

Normal hearing means that a sound made at a particular frequency (Hertz) 500Hz, 1000Hz or 2,000Hz, for example, can be heard 50% of the time when it is between 0-19 decibels(measures of loudness).

Class 1: Very mild/mild loss means sound is heard when it is between 20-40dbs (decibels). 20-30% of the ability to hear is lost. Hearing speech is rated at good to fair.

Class 2: Moderate loss means sound is heard when it is between 41-55dbs. 30-40% of hearing is lost. Hearing speech is rated at fair to poor.

Class 3: Moderate/severe loss means sound is heard when it is between 56-70dbs. 45-50% of hearing is lost. Hearing speech is rated at poor.

Class 4: Severe loss means sound is heard when it is between 71-90dbs. More than 50% of hearing is lost. Hearing speech is rated at very poor.

Class 5: Profound loss means sound is heard when it is more than 90 dbs. There is no functional hearing. No speech is heard.

2

THEIR FEELINGS, YOUR FEELIINGS

The majority of people with hearing loss live and spend most of their time with those who hear. They work in environments that depend on hearing noises and voices. In many cases, being with those that hear makes it possible for the deaf to carry out common tasks more safely or efficiently. For example, many people need to use friends who hear to alert them when smoke alarms go off, to make phone calls for them, or to notify them when someone is calling them.

However, it is both difficult and exhausting for people who are deaf to understand others in our hearing culture. Many people with hearing losses need to see the speaker's lips in order to lip-read, and watch facial and body gestures in order to fully understand the message. Those with normal hearing often don't speak clearly, finish sentences, or look at the person being addressed.

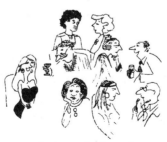

Party or nightmare?

Often people who are hard of hearing are treated as if they not only cannot hear but cannot see, think, or feel. They are ignored by people who hear.

Deaf people report that they experience the greatest communication with others who have hearing losses. They confirm and support each other's experiences and identities as individuals with a common linguistic and cultural history. This sense of support is a strong characteristic of the deaf culture.

THEIR FEELINGS

anxiety: I would like to be a part of the conversation, but I don't know what is being said around me; I don't know if I am safe where I am, if I can't hear the alarm, phone, footsteps, or oncoming car.

anger: I don't appreciate jokes about deafness; I have a hearing loss. Shouting at me won't change that.

loneliness: I have difficulty keeping up with the conversation when I can't lipread, watch signs or gestures, or read the message. I feel sad because I am ignored when I'm with others who hear.

embarrassment: I can get embarrassed when I misread or misinterpret the message and locate the cat when they asked for some cake. Just because I am deaf doesn't mean I know sign language.

fatigue: I am exhausted trying to keep up with reading people's lips when they speak, guessing who will speak next, and what each person will be speaking about throughout each conversation every day.

YOUR FEELINGS

anxiety: I don't know what else I can do to communicate besides speaking.

I don't know sign.

I don't know how to behave.

I don't know if he or she understands me.

I will probably say or do something to offend him or her.

Trying to talk to a deaf person is too hard for me.

disbelief: He could understand me if I shout or really exaggerate my words.

She is pretending to be deaf.

If I can't see the disability, it's hard to believe it exists.

fear: I could get it.

I couldn't survive being deaf.

I prefer not to talk to a deaf person.

If he or she can read my lips, can they read my mind?

empathy: Their lives must be difficult.

I want to help.

I'll try to show them my lips and speak slowly and clearly.

enjoyment: This person is a lot of fun to be around.

Learning and using sign language is fun.

There may be as many feelings about deafness or hearing loss as there are variations on the degree and nature of the hearing loss itself. The intensity of your feelings may depend on your relationship with a person who is hard of hearing. Reaching out to prevent a stranger on a street corner from stepping into traffic because the person cannot hear a car's horn might increase your anxiety about deafness, or it might stimulate your compassion. (Of course, if the situation were reversed, and you were assisted by someone deaf because you did not notice the oncoming car, your appreciation for her capabilities might increase.)

On the other hand, if you are a relative, or a friend of a deaf person, or one who is hard of hearing, your feelings may be more intense. Sometimes, trying to communicate something important or meaningful is as frustrating and isolating as two people trying to speak to each other through an impregnable glass window: the sound cannot be heard, just the frustration and disappointment seen and felt in each attempt.

3

MANNERS THAT MATTER; BOTH SIDES

Most people depend on conversation as their way of meeting or relating to others and making friends. Speaking and listening are very effective and safe methods to communicate with others and to find out if they are open to relating back.

For some people, hearing loss interferes with the ability to distinguish speech or to speak clearly. Because the disability is invisible, other people do not think to use alternate forms of communication such as tapping them on the arm for attention or writing messages down. As a result many people with significant hearing losses are left out of conversations, and therefore miss the opportunity to make friends or even simple contact.

This experience of social isolation can be devasting if it is not balanced by a supportive network of family and friends who use other techniques to communicate or who have this disability. Here are some easy methods you can use when you are around those with hearing impairments:

YOUR MANNERS

In general

1. Remember that this is a person with a disability, not a disabled person.

2. Focus on what someone can do, and offer assistance only

where it is obviously needed.

3. Allow extra time for someone with a hearing impairment to interpret what you say or to communicate with you.

4. When you want to attract someone's attention, tap on the arm. Do not poke or grab. If you are at a distance, wave. If someone with a hearing loss is looking down while reading or writing for example, knock on the desk. If it is an emergency, turn the lights on and off.

5. Let the deaf person know when you are entering or leaving the room.

6. Remember, some handicaps are more invisible than others. Some can be hidden, some cannot.

Communication

1. Look at the person to whom you are talking. Do not turn away or block your face while you are talking. Remember the person needs to see your expressions and your lips.

2. Speak clearly, calmly, and slowly. Do not over exaggerate your words. It will make lipreading much more difficult. Most people only get 30-35% of the message through lipreading as it is.

3. Speak in your normal voice. Shouting will not improve their

hearing. Many people with hearing loss can hear some sound which helps them with lipreading.

4. Listen closely. Someone with a hearing impairment may have difficulty articulating words. Do not pretend to understand what you do not.

5. Be prepared to repeat your sentence. Feel free to ask them to repeat theirs.

6. If they do not understand what you are saying, write it down. Ask them to write their message down as well.

7. Use normal gestures while you talk if they enhance your communication. Do not let the intensity of the subject matter make you gesture wildly, or forget to speak clearly .

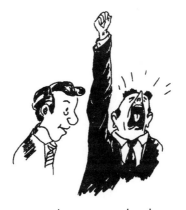

No need to raise your hand at me.

8. If you do not know Sign Language, do not invent your own.

9. If you know American Sign Language, ask your companion if he or she knows signing before using it. Signing is not a naturally developed instinct: it is a learned skill.

10. Learn a few signs in American Sign Language. It is easy and fun. Learn to fingerspell the alphabet.

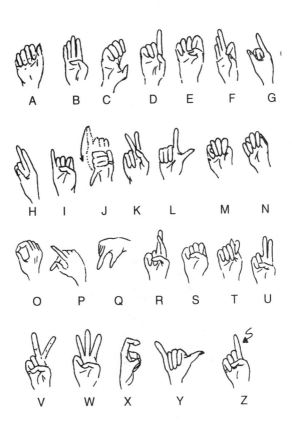

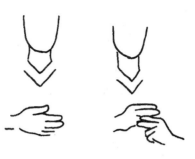

MY NAME (IS)

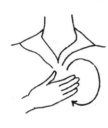

PLEASE

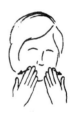

THANK YOU

REPEAT

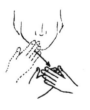

GOOD

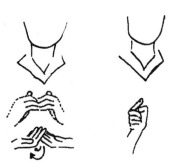

HOW (ARE) YOU?

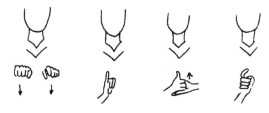

CAN I HELP YOU?

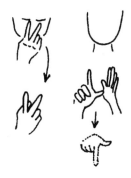

SEE (YOU) LATER

THEIR MANNERS

1. Allow extra time for people without disabilities to understand you. They are not used to your way of talking or gesturing.

2. Be prepared to repeat or write down what you said. Ask them to repeat or write down what they said if you do not understand them.

3. Speak calmly, clearly, and slowly. It is not necessary (nor polite) to shout or overexaggerate your words. And they probably can't lipread at all.

4. Use gestures, pictures, facial expressions to enhance your message. Do not assume they know sign language just because you do.

5. Teach them some sign language.

Everybody's responsibility

Try to communicate effectively and frequently with a friend and or a relative, with anyone who happens to have hearing problems. Make an effort to take deaf people out of their routines, just for a break. Accompany them on trips or errands when they need the help of a hearing person. Translate movies or plays, interpret directions, take notes during lectures.

Take a class with your friends in sign language. It is a lot of fun. And quite useful in loud environments or places where you don't want others to know what you are saying.

Use American Sign Language as a way of including everyone in our multicultural world: this would be significant step in acknowledging people with special needs as a part of our community, and not outside of it.

4

SEEKING A DIAGNOSIS

Because hearing loss involves degrees of impairment, and can be acquired at any stage including birth, it is a disability that frequently goes undetected. Many people with mild hearing losses have learned to compensate for their difficulties without professional help or assistive devices such as hearing aids. In some people who have other disabilities such as attention deficit disorder, cerebral palsy, or mental retardation, a hearing impairment can be missed.

A diagnosis of a hearing impairment is made by a specialist in hearing disorders called an audiologist. The audiologist may also use test results from an otologist, a specialist in ear diseases; or an otolaryngologist, a specialist in all the structures of the ear, nose, and throat.

The most frequently used hearing tests include impedance testing, pure tone assessment, and speech hearing assessment.

Impedance testing

The impedance testing involves a probe placed in the ear allowing varying degrees of sounds and air pressures to be sent into the ear. It is not an uncomfortable test unless there is an ear infection. This test checks for conductive hearing loss.

Pure-tone hearing assessment

In this procedure, sounds are presented at different frequencies and volumes through speakers, headphones, or small devices placed behind the ear while the client stands in a soundproof booth. This test measures both conductive and sensorineural hearing loss.

Speech hearing assessment

During this assessment, a list of words is read to the client in a soundproof booth. The client indicates that he or she hears the words by repeating the words or by pointing to pictures representing the words if the client cannot speak. The reader may vary the loudness of the words or ask the person in the booth to discriminate between similar sounding words.

Hearing tests are modified for those not able to follow the standard hearing tests. For example, some people with severe mental retardation may require preparation for the tests, such as being rewarded for responding to the sounds. This modified test is called the Tangible Reinforcement Operant Conditioning Audiometry (TROCA).

Infants or those people with severe disabilities such as profound mental retardation may be given the Brain Stem Audiometry (ABR) or the Heart Rate Response Audiometry (HRRA). These tests require no active response on the patient's part. Brain and heart activity are monitored as sounds are produced at different frequencies and volumes.

Temporary hearing loss

Some hearing losses such those caused by excessive ear wax or re-occuring ear infections are temporary and can be treated at the source of the problem: that is, removal of ear wax; medication to cure the infection; or drainage of the fluid building up in the ear. In some cases, a tube may be surgically placed in the eardrum to create continuous draining for a period of up to two years.

Permanent hearing loss

Permanent hearing losses may be improved by surgery to correct malformations, or to repair injured ear structures such as with cochlear(inner ear) implants.

Hearing aids

Hearing aids are commonly used by people who have hearing loss. Hearing aids amplify sounds and broaden the range of tones. Those who have difficulty with volume alone respond well to the aids. Those with hearing loss that includes distortion of sound as well may need many lessons to adjust to the use of a hearing aid.

ALTO Z HEARING AID BY BELTONE

SIEMENS BTE AID
FITS BEHIND THE EAR

Hearing aids come in many varieties. Some are worn behind the ear and have a tube that leads into the ear canal sending vibrations. For those who have normal hearing in one ear, two aids are used; one aid sends sound from the affected ear to the receiving aid in the normal hearing ear.

Hearing aids may contain pocket controls that can adjust volume and tone. Aids can also be worn on the body. Body aids are sturdier, function over a wide range of frequencies, and are therefore suitable for young children or those with severe or profound mental retardation. Personal microphone systems called FM's are used in classrooms to reduce background noise: the teacher wears a microphone that leads to the student's earphone.

Although hearing aids open up a world of sound to those with hearing loss, they require getting used to and can be very inconvenient to maintain. They require batteries, and regular monitoring for replacement. They can squeal or whistle when not correctly inserted or disconnected. Hearing aids can take time to fit comfortably. Some aids need repeated repairs due to electronic malfunctions.

CHOOSING A SUPPORT SYSTEM

The impact a hearing loss has on any individual depends on many factors such as the degree of hearing loss, the age at which it occured, and on the individual's ability to compensate or rely on environmental supports to compensate for the loss. For example, adults who have already developed language skills and knowledge of the environment may have psychological difficulty in adjusting to a hearing loss at work and at home. People born without hearing will have had no auditory contact with hearing people and will need special assistance from family,friends, and teachers to acquire essential language and life experience skills.

Therefore, in selecting professionals, schools, and programs, it is important to keep the needs of the individual as the focus of the support system. The support system should be developed around individual strengths, needs, and abilities to compensate for the hearing loss.

DOCTORS

Medical treatment includes surgery, as well as physical, occupational and/or speech therapy. For those born with medical conditions that accompany a hearing loss such as cranial or facial deformities or cerebral palsy, therapy can begin while they are infants in order to correct the condition or minimize the impact of the physical disabilities on later functioning.

When choosing a doctor, look for empathy, knowledge of the disabilities involved, experience, and the doctor's ability to assist you in accessing additional community resources.

SCHOOLS

If you child is diagnosed with deafness during infancy, educational programs start between the ages of one and three. The primary focus of these programs is to assist you, the parents, expecially if you have normal hearing, to adjust to your child's disability and teach you how to provide the necessary stimulation and develop communication skills within the family that include the child.

Children usually enter the school system at age five. Approximately one third of these children will attend residential schools. Other children will attend special schools. In the special schools, the students will experience the benefits and support of the deaf culture. They will be with others who share their disability and can identify with the difficulties of living in a hearing world. For example, those children with severe hearing losses or who are deaf will need to learn English as other students would a foreign language for reading, speech reading, or speaking. It is a frustrating and difficult process since they cannot hear speech articulated as children who hear do.

Students in special schools will be exposed to information about people who are deaf or hard of hearing who have achieved personal and professional successes. They are also more likely to learn of special youth enrichment and leadership programs made possible by the National Association of the Deaf such as the Junior NAD and Youth Leadership Camp (see Appendix for addresses).

Children with hearing loss are able to meet the challenges of a regular school environment if provided extra support. Plans for these students can include a classroom interpreter, tutoring, speech therapy, and notetakers. Technical aids, including hearing aids, cochlear implants, or personal microphones, can accompany the student. Although they attend special classes for some part of the day, these children are able to develop friendships with other children who do not have disabilities. In some instances, students may need to leave school early each day to go to a separate therapy service.

When choosing a school, you may wish to consider the staff's philosophies toward the role of education, community integration, and quality of life for children with hearing loss. Compare their views with yours regarding the kind of adults these children will become: how they will fit into society, live, and work.

Find out the degree to which the school emphasizes vocational training vs. basic academics; signing vs. speechreading/speaking. Educating students who are deaf with an emphasis in oral communication vs. combining manual and oral language has been a controversy of significant intensity for over a hundred years. One philosophy strongly advocated by educators such as Alexander Graham Bell suggests that all people learn to use audible speech. These educators feel deaf students need to learn to communicate with speech and speechreading in order to live and work in the hearing community.

The opposing philosophy, articulated by Edward Miner Gallaudet, educator and father of the founder of Gallaudet University, is that people who are deaf do best by using both a manual and oral system of communication.Schools vary in their approach and emphasize their philosophy in their curriculums.

Also, find out where their students go after graduation – vocational training, day programs, or out on their own to obtain jobs and integrate into their own neighborhoods. Decide what is best for your child. The best schools will design individualized plans which take into account each student's preferences, strengths, and outside supports (family, friends, other social services).

It is also recommended that you research the school's standing on service delivery and quality with the regional Board of Education. If the school has a residential program, check with the licensing state agency, or the National Association of the Deaf (for addresses and phone/TDD numbers, see Appendix) to ensure the schools are up to date with their inspections and compliance measures.

Many deaf or hearing impaired students go on to attend colleges. Some attend regular colleges with similar special supports they received in high school. Others attend colleges especially developed for deaf students such as Gallaudet University or National Technical Institute for the Deaf. There are over 100 additional community and technical schools as well.

WORK

People who are hard of hearing or deaf compete for and obtain the same jobs as those without hearing difficulties. They become scientists, salespeople, dancers, artists, and actors. For example, the National Theatre of the Deaf is comprised of a group of actors who are deaf. There are support organizations for professionals who are deaf in fields of teaching, social work, and small business (for addresses and phone/TDD numbers, see Appendix).

5

LIVING WITH HEARING LOSS: A DAY IN A LIFE

Sign language can be traced back to early civilizations in which forms of sign language were used prior to the development of verbal language. Deafness and use of signing was acknowledged in ancient Hebrew and Greek cultures according to texts such as the Talmud and works of Plato and Aristotle.

During the early 1500's, Pedro Ponce de Leon of Spain, a monk, was one of the first advocates for deaf people. He taught a deaf man, previously turned away because of his deafness, to read , even to speak partially, in order to be accepted as a postulant in the Benedictine Monastery in San Salvador. He was the first recorded individual to use signing to teach students who were deaf. He and other monks had been using signing as a means of communication in monasteries where they had taken vows of silence.

During the 1600's, schools were established for students who were deaf in Europe. Some countries, such as Germany, only taught oral communication, while other countries, such as France, taught the combined method. Thomas Hopkins Gallaudet, an American, went to France to learn sign language. He encouraged a French teacher, Laurent Clerc to come to America to open the first school for the deaf. Today it is known as the American School for the Deaf, and is located in Hartford, Connecticut.

Despite the few individuals with hearing who are noted in the history of the deaf culture, most hearing cultures have treated the deaf as freaks. People with deafness were punished for having this disability. Because deaf children did not learn spoken language they were treated as though they had mental retardation and frequently locked away in asylums with beggars, prostitutes, and people with mental illnesses.

Conditions are improving for deaf people. There are a large number of advocacy and educational programs available to those with hearing impairments including the National Association of the Deaf Legal Defense Fund (NADLDF). The NADLDF advocates for the legal rights for those who are deaf or hard of hearing in situations such as education, work, and health care.

In 1990, the Americans with Disabilities Act was passed as a Federal Civil Rights Law. It provides for equal opportunity, full participation, independent living, and self-sufficiency for all people with disabilities in employment and life. The law has already helped many people achieve access to jobs, housing, public buildings (such as clinics, voting booths, schools, and churches), and transportation that were previously inaccessible or unattainable. For example, previous to this law supporting accessibility, people with physical disabilities were barred from participation in whatever their disabilities inhibited. People with hearing impairments could not worship or attend regular schools because they were not able to hear the messages or lessons.

ADA has required assistive devices such as closed caption (spoken words printed out, for instance on a television screen), or that interpretors be made available. Electronic road and highway signs that report traffic conditions are one way the government accomodates those who cannot tune into the radio stations for traffic reports.

While the law can mandate and enforce structural and policy based regulations for accessibility, it cannot institute a change in peoples' attitudes. In this area, people with disabilities still struggle for the right to be treated equally and with dignity.

Karen

Karen is a 22- year- old woman who was diagnosed with moderate hearing loss as an infant. She could acknowledge sounds, but they were muffled. The hearing aids she wore helped only modestly to increase her ability to pick up sound. Although she attended regular schools, Karen participated in special tutoring during class periods, was given written notes of class instruction, and written tests instead of oral exams. Karen's parents enrolled her in special programs to learn sign language and to receive speech therapy. Karen went on to college to become an occupational therapist.

As an adult Karen spends her work day with those that hear, and most of her free time with friends who don't. Like other young adults, Karen loves music and turns up her car radio on the way to work so that she can feel the vibrations. Karen's employer has provided a telephone equipped with a telecommunication device for the deaf (TDD) for her use. Alarms have lights that blink for emergencies.

Although some procedures have been modified to accomodate Karen's difficulty, such as not using the overhead paging system to notify Karen of her patients' arrivals, phone calls or meetings, co-workers still forget their manners when they are with Karen. These courtesies include facing Karen when they are talking to her, touching her arm when they want her attention, and including her in their conversation. They also seem to think that because she cannot hear them, it is all right to talk about her in her presence.

Theodore

Ted, 31 years old, was diagnosed with mental retardation at the age of two and admitted to a state institution at age three by his overwhelmed parents. According to Ted's parents, Ted was unresponsive to others and his environment – his parents felt he had not bonded with them and that they could not provide the level of care he seemed to need.

As an adolescent, Ted was diagnosed with a severe hearing loss. Perhaps in part, due to the lack of awareness of his family about hearing loss and their not knowing how to adjust to Ted's limitations, the stimulation essential to his development was never provided as an infant and toddler. This lack of stimulation may have exacerbated the developmental delays later diagnosed as mental retardation.

Being diagnosed with mental retardation, Ted was never accorded services normally provided to children who are deaf. As a result, Ted performed at the level expected for someone with moderate mental retardation.

At 21, Ted was admitted into a private agency's residential

program in a group home setting. Counselors who provided Ted with individual attention recognized Ted's ability to learn new skills including sign language. He was able to make friends with others in his programs both at home and work. With special vocational training, Ted now works as part of a work crew in a large department store.

Jarrod

Jarrod was born to parents who were deaf. He attended a regular school until he was 4. He was diagnosed with a moderate hearing loss and was admitted to a school for the deaf. Hearing aids improved his ability to pick up and distinguish sounds and speech therapy assisted Jarrod to use spoken language in communicating in addition to sign language. Although he could have hidden his disability, his exposure to and support by the deaf culture both at home and in school led to a strong sense of confidence and identity about being hard of hearing.

When Jarrod graduated from a regular college and applied to a graduate program to study child development and teaching, he was rejected based on his disability. The school felt his inability to hear would pose a safety threat to children under his supervision.

As a result of legal action demonstrating the school's violation of the ADA, and advocacy from professionals who reported on deaf teachers' abilities to teach safely and effectively, Jarrod was admitted to the program.

Kenneth

Kenneth scored well on tests, and played varsity football and baseball. Against the recommendation of his high school guidance teacher who advised him to seek out trade schools because of his disability, Kenneth applied for an was accepted to an ivy league university.

This is Kenneth's first day of classes. As he enters his classroom, he quietly acknowledges the interpreter assigned to his class to help him understand the lecture. He takes a seat and greets a classmate who does not understand him. After several more attempts on Kenneth's part, the other student simples waves "hi" and turns to chat with other students who have formed a circle to the side. Kenneth cannot see their gestures nor read their lips. Not knowing what they are saying or if it is a private conversation, Kenneth decides not to join them. He looks straight ahead.

Before class begins, the professor points out the interpreter to the class, makes statements to support the integration of the disabled, and explains how Kenneth requires special assistance. Kenneth feels like a sideshow.

During the lecture, the buzzer signals the end of class, his classmates bound out of their seats and out of the classroom. Kenneth, who cannot hear the bell, takes his cue from watching the others and follows them out into the hallway toward their next class, alone.

Heather Whitestone

Heather Whitestone's role model was Helen Keller. Heather

became the first deaf Miss America, a triumph based on her mother's and her own refusal to base her life on a handicap instead of on her own abilities and dreams. She learned to talk, later to sign. She is at home in the deaf culture as well as the hearing culture.

A NOTE ABOUT FAMILIES

Having a deaf child requires parents and siblings to examine, and perhaps significantly adjust, their values about deafness. For parents who are deaf, the adjustment may be far easier. However, it probably means special services, special schools, endless trips to adjust, repair, or replace hearing aids or assistive communication devices. It may also include special medical attention if your child is born with other physical conditions (cranial or facial deformities). Entire family structures are altered; finances can be drained.

As your child develops, you and other family members must adapt your ways of living to meet the needs of the child. You need to learn new ways to communicate with and teach your child. You must learn to be guardian, an advocate, and sometimes an activist for your child's rights to receive adequate care and equal opportunity. Siblings must adjust to receiving less attention and perhaps greater responsibilities within the household or in protecting a brother or sister with hearing loss when out in the neighborhood.

Even into adulthood, the person with a hearing impairment may require continued support and advocacy from the family.

You may find it necessary to continue to act as guardian when other disabilities are present such as mental retardation. In such a case, you will be required to make decisions about medical treatment, finances, and where the person will live and work.

It is also true that to have a family member who is deaf or hard of hearing can be very rewarding: it can deepen your bonds and make relationships more meaningful and appreciated.

Having a friend who is deaf can be rewarding for the same reasons. To share the problems and challenges of a friend with a disability can bring depth and humor and an abiding affection to your relationship. It brings the joy of deeper personal insight, as well as a deeper understanding of people with disabilities.

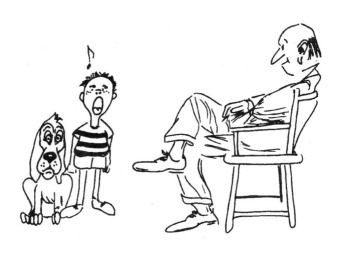

Deafness: advantages in family life.

6

RESOURCES: FUNDING; TRAINING; JOB OPPORTUNITIES; HOUSING; APPLIANCES; DIET AND EXERCISE

Special services, assistive equipment, and advocacy support are more accessible today than in the past. Laws such as the ADA are being enforced to provide equal opportunity and reasonable accomodation in communities. Yet, in dealing with disabilities, advocates acknowledge that the three "P's" are still required: knowledge of Policies and laws that protect the rights of people with disabilities; Patience while negotiating through the kinks in the systems; and Persistence to insist you get the resources you need.

ALWAYS REMEMBER TO:

Write down:

- the date and time of contact
- whether it was in person or on the phone
- phone number (and extension)
- name and title of the person with whom you talked
- stated agreements or conditions to receive services
- dates to follow-up on stated agreements or conditions

Having this information on record can mean the difference between the social service agency providing what was agreed to in the conversation and denying any record of your approaching the agency at all.

BE PERSISTENT AND POLITE

Do not give in or give up. Remember the person you are talking to has the service or information you need. Acknowledge that you do not know the systems as well as the person you are talking to. Request detailed verbal and written information regarding the system as well as the qualifications of the person rendering the assistance. Don't be afraid or shy about asking for whatever help and assistance you need .

SOCIAL SERVICE RESOURCES AND FUNDING

It is best to start at the national level to get a listing of all the resources, training, and advocacy assistance available to you nationally and where you live. The National Association of the Deaf can provide such information and support (for address and phone/TDD, see Appendix).

TRAINING AND JOB OPPORTUNITIES

People who are hard of hearing or deaf are capable of pursuing all of the same careers as those who can hear, with a few

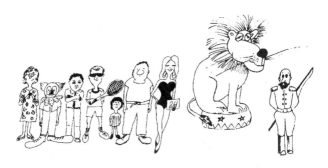

A person who is deaf can have many professions.

exceptions. Naturally, they can not perform jobs that rely heavily on hearing such as a radio disk jockey, telephone operator, or choir master. People who are deaf have become almost everything else, though – dancers, musicians, scientists, teachers, lawyers,or whatever else interests them to become. This includes football players (the football huddle was invented for deaf players at Gallaudet College in the 1890's).

The deaf culture is comprised of a strong network of social, financial, advocacy, and educational support. Perhaps the largest organization within this culture is the National Association of the Deaf (NAD). The NAD serves as a warehouse of information and publishes books, journals, and newsletters such as *The Deaf American*.

The American Athletic Association of the Deaf operates national sports competitions. Every four years an International Olympics is hosted by deaf sponsors.

After years of discrimination due to misconceptions about the disability, deaf entrepreneurs developed the National Fraternal Society offering life and medical insurance to the deaf. The society also sponsors social events for the deaf.

Special schools have been founded just for those who are deaf, including Gallaudet University in Washington, DC and Rochester Institute of Technology in Rochester, NY.

Of notable acclaim is the National Theatre of the Deaf. Started by psychologist Dr. Edna Levine, David Hays, Mary Switzer, and the Department of Health, Education, and Welfare administrator Dr. Boyce Williams, the National Theatre of the

Deaf tours nationally and has performed on Broadway and at Lincoln Center in New York City. Performances have been broadcasted on national television. The National Theatre of the Deaf is comprised of actors who can and cannot hear. Actors on stage are deaf and use sign. Hearing actors narrate or fill in dialogue, but the deaf actors rely on exaggerated facial expression, expressive body language, and sign language. "Sign language is an art form, says Laine Dyer, spokesperson for the Theatre of the Deaf. "Deaf actors are natural born actors."

Actor Robert DeMayo, who is deaf, says, "I'm not a deaf actor. I'm an actor who happens to be deaf. I use my eyes a lot. My eyes are my ears."

This acting group has made tremendous inroads into increasing the awareness of the general public about deafness, and about the abilities of the population of and culture of people with deafness.

HEARING DOGS

Hearing dogs are now available for people who are deaf. PAWS (Paws with a Cause) offers trained dogs for the hearing impaired or physically disabled, to enhance their owners' abilities. Hearing dogs take about four months to train and can help their owners by alerting them to beeper and telephone, the doorbell or the cry of a child. PAWS has placed more than 900 hearing dogs since 1979. Ninety-five percent of hearing dogs have been rescued from animal shelters. For more information, call 1-800-253-PAWS.

Communication aids

Hearing aids, signal devices, TDD's (telecommunications devices for the deaf), TTY's(teletype devices), and telecaption decoders are electronic communication aids.

Hearing aids serve to enhance sound and the range of tones for the wearer.

Signal devices are blinking lights or vibrations that replace the sounds of an alarm clock, fire alarm, child crying, telephone or door bell.

TDD's, telecommunication devices, are essentially processors with a modem attached. The handset is placed on the keyboard in a similar way to a modem. As the person communicates through typing his or her message, he or she can read the caller's responses across the screen. Most businesses and all government agencies are required by the ADA to have TDD's.

Telecaption decoders are the closed caption option now built into most televisions. Closed captions are like subtitles.

"In the near future, however, people will be going online with computers, and as the world moves more and more in the direction of computers, deaf people will become indistiguishable from hearing people," believes David Hays, founding artistic director of the National Theatre of the Deaf.

Communication methods

People who are deaf or hard of hearing have many ways to

communicate. Using the American Sign Language (ASL), other-wsie known as signing, is most commonly used among those who have learned to sign at school or through special training. The language uses hand motion and position with a different syntax and grammar than spoken English.

Fingerspelling, which follows a manual alphabet, is used for proper nouns or words for which there are no signs.

When sign language and fingerspelling incorporate the English language and follow English word order, it is called "pidgin" sign English (PSE). This is used occasionally to assist young students to learn English.

Speechreading or lipreading is a necessary but highly unreli-able method for people who are deaf when someone is talking to them, since only approximately 30% of English sounds are distinguishable. Many people combine the context of the conver-sation with gestures from the speaker. Speechreading is easier for those who have some degree of hearing.

DIET AND EXERCISE

All people require healthy diet and regular exercise. For those people with other physical conditions that accompany hearing losses, exercise is particularly important in order not to complicate their health with obesity that can lead to heart dis-ease, adult diabetes, or cardiovascular disorders.

7

FIX YOUR ATTITUDE, YOUR HOME, AND YOUR COMMUNITY

Making your home accessible to visitors who have disabilities is one major step toward embracing others with differences and including them in your life. Accomodations are easy to make and very often increase our own convenience at home. "Reasonable accomodation," according to the ADA, "means making adjustments to architectural and procedural barriers that are readily achievable."

EXPERIMENT

Turn on your television to a program you have been looking forward to watching. Now, turn the volume all the way down. Try to follow the story line without the sound. Ask yourself how you feel when you cannot understand what the actors are saying, especially when you are not sure of the context of the situation or conversation.

Making your home accessible to a visitor who is deaf means being sensitive to the experience of not hearing and using the manners recommended in the chapter "Manners That Matter: Both Sides."

When out in the community, shopping, or eating at a restaurant, try the exercise you did at home by closing off your ears. One important step toward making your community more accessible would be to encourage the store or restaurant owners to make accomodations" that are "readily achievable" just as you have done at home. Encourage cinemas to include more films with closed caption. Remind them that people with disabilities are customers, too.

Speak up when you see the injustice of inaccessibility for anyone, but begin with your own attitudes and behavior. Learn some ASL,, so you can communicate with a deaf friend, relative, or newcomer in your life today.

8

SELECTED DISORDERS

Deafness is a separate problem, just as blindness or any other anomaly that occurs as a genetic or birth defect or is acquired later on. But because it is so often overlooked when other problems are present, this is a partial listing of disorders with which deafness is sometimes associated.

Sensory aphasia

Aphasia is defined as an inability to use symbols for communication. It involves a partial or total lack of speech resulting from injury to the brain. Children who are born with or acquire sensory aphasia show an inability to understand or use language, and a poor memory for learning language. Some significant signs of sensory aphasia include use of jargon or scribble speech, repetition of words without association of meaning, and infrequent vocalizations.

Sensory aphasia is difficult to determine in some cases as it is accompanied by different levels of intelligence, social behavior, personality styles, and degrees of hearing impairment. All of these factors serve to impact on the child's functioning to varying degrees. Most of these children are able to make friends and engage in social activities. They communicate by gestures rather than by speech. However, they require special education for language development.

Some children with deafness do not respond accurately to testing for sensory aphasia and are put in classes for the deaf that do not address the aphasia.

Cleft palate

Cleft palate is a split or opening that separates the structures of the mouth. Impairments range from a slight notch in the lip to complete separation of the soft and hard palates, to a complete absence of a particular anatomical structure in the mouth. Causes include maternal diseases, bleeding, acccidents, illnesses, taking certain medications, or poor nutrition during pregnancy.

Damage to the oral structures may include malformed auditory anatomy as well such as the eustachian tube, auditory nerve, or muscles around the ear. Conductive hearing loss can result ranging from mild to moderate.

Mental retardation

Mental retardation can be present at birth or occur any time during development through infancy, childhood, and adolescence; that is, before age 18. It is defined by the significant limitations someone has in functioning and adapting both to daily routines and new challenges during his or her life. IQ is a factor, but not the only one.

Some people with mental retardation go to regular high schools, graduate, and get jobs. Some require assistance with working and living. Some need more assistance in dressing, feeding themselves, and toileting.

Many people with mental retardation also have some degree of hearing impairment due to the malformation of auditory or nerve structures.

APPENDIX

SOURCES FOR HELP

Alexander Graham Bell Association for the Deaf
3417 Volta Place, NE
Washington, DC 20007
(202)337-5220 V/TTY

American Deafness and Rehabilitation
PO Box 251554
Little Rock, AR 72225
(501)868-8850 V/TTY

American Society for Deaf Children
2848 Arden Way, Suite 210
Sacramento, CA 95825-1373
(800)942-ASDC V/TTY

National Association of the Deaf (NAD)
Junior NAD, Youth Leadership Camp (YLC)
American Association of the Deaf-Blind
814 Thayer Avenue
Silver Spring, MD 20910
(301)588-6545 TTY

American Society of Deaf Social Workers
1306 Morningside Drive
Silver Spring, MD 20904
(202)373-7215

Association of Late-Deafened Adults
PO Box 641763
Chicago, IL 60664
(815)459-5741 TTY

Deaf and Hard of Hearing Entrepreneurs Council
817 Silver Spring Ave, Suite 305-F
Silver Spring, MD 20910-4617
(301)587-8596 TTY

Gallaudet University
National Information Center on Deafness
800 Florida Ave. NE
Washington, DC 20002
(202)651-5000 V/TTY

Helen Keller National Center for Deaf-Blind Youths and Adults
111 Middle Neck Road
Sandy Point, NY 11050
(516)944-8900 V/TTY

National Black Deaf Advocates, Inc.
Pamela Lloy, President
1415 Gardenwood Drive
College Park, GA 30349
(404)997-1489

National Technical Institute for the Deaf
52 Lomb Memorial Drive
PO Box 9887/LBJ Bldg.

Rochester, NY 14623-5604
(716)475-2181 TTY • (716)475-6400 V

National Theatre of the Deaf
5 West Main St.
PO Box 659
Chester, CT 06412
(203)526-4974 TTY • (203)526-4971 V

Telecommunications for the Deaf, Inc.
8719 Colesville Road, Suite 300
Silver Spring, MD 20910
(301)589-3006 TTY • (301)589-3786 V

National Association fo the Deaf Legal Defense Fund
800 Florida Ave. NE
PO Box 2304
Washington, DC. 20002
(202)651-5343 TTY/V

American Athletic Association of the Deaf
3916 Lantern Drive
Silver Spring, MD 20902
(301)942-4042

American School for the Deaf
139 N. Main Street
West Hartford, CT 06107
(203)727-1300

REFERENCES AND RECOMMENDED READING

Cohen, Leah Hager, *Train Go Sorry: Inside a Deaf World,* Houghton Mifflin Company, New York. 1994

Deafness: A Fact Sheet. National Information Center on Deafness, National Association of the Deaf. Gallaudet College, Washington, DC. 1984.

Holvet, Jennifer F., Helmstetter, Edwin. *Medical Problems of Students with Special Needs: A Guide for Educators,* College-Hill Press. A division of Little, Brown and Company, Boston, MA, 1989.

Communicate! Sign Language You Can Learn, American School for the Deaf, West Hartford, CT, 1994.

Maloff, Chalda, *Business and Social Etiquette with Disabled People,* Charles C. Thomas, Springfield, IL, 1988.

Communicating With People Who Have A Hearing Loss. Alexander Graham Bell Association for the Deaf, Washington, DC, 1994.

Riekehof, Lottie L, *The Joy of Signing,* Gospel Publishing House. Springfield, MA, 1993.

Davis, H., and Silverman, R.S., *Hearing and Deafness* (4th ed.)

Holt, Rinehart and Winston, New York, 1978.

Spradley, Thomas S., and Spradley, James P., *Deaf Like Me.* Univ. of California Press, New York, 1972.

Meadow, Kathryn P. *Deafness and Child Development.* Univ. of California Press. Berkeley, CA. 1980.

Hardman, M., et al, eds., *Human Exceptionality: Society, School, and Family,* Allyn and Bacon, Simon and Schuster, Needham Heights, MA, 1993.

McGinnis, M. Aphasic *Children: Identification and Education* by the Association Method, Alexander Graham Bell Association for the Deaf, Washington, DC, 1963.

Westlake, H. and Rutherford, D., *Cleft Palate,* Prentice-Hall, Englewood, NJ, 1966.

Mindel, E., MD, and Vernon, M. MD, *They Grow in Silence: The Deaf Child and His Family,* National Association of the Deaf, Silverspring, MD, 1971.

Winefield, R. *Never the Twain Shall Meet: The Communications Debate,* Gallaudet University Press, Washington, DC, 1987.

Keller, Helen Adams, *The Story of My Life,* Grosset & Dunlop, NY, 1902.

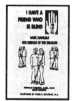
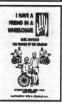
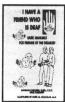